Table of Contents

PREVIEW

Chemotherapy is the use of drugs to destroy cancer cells. This type of cancer treatment works by keeping cancer cells from growing, dividing, and making more cells.

Chemotherapy can be used as a treatment for many different cancers. Your doctor may refer to chemotherapy as standard chemotherapy, traditional chemotherapy, or cytotoxic chemotherapy.

The word "chemotherapy" ("chemo") is often used when referring to medicines or drugs that treat cancer. But, not all drugs used to treat cancer work in the same way. Traditional or standard chemotherapy uses drugs that are cytotoxic, meaning they can kill tumor cells. If your treatment plan includes traditional or standard chemotherapy, knowing how it works and what to expect can often help you prepare for treatment and make informed decisions about your care.

A healthy body constantly replaces cells through a process of dividing, growing, and dying. When cancer occurs, cells reproduce uncontrollably and do not die when they should.

As a part of the body produces more and more of these abnormal cells, they start to occupy the space that useful cells previously took up.

Chemotherapy drugs interfere with a cancer cell's ability to divide and reproduce. Drugs vary in how they work. Different drugs attack cancer cells at different phases in the cell life cycle.

Treatment can attack rapidly dividing cells throughout the body or only specific substances or parts of cancer cells.

BREAKFAST

1. Strata

Prep Time: 20 Minutes

Cook Time: 55 Minutes

Servings: 12

Ingredients

- 2 tablespoons olive oil plus more for the baking dish
- 1 16-ounce French baguette cubed
- 1 onion thinly sliced
- 1 teaspoon salt divided
- 1 teaspoon black pepper divided
- 1 8-ounce container sliced baby bella mushrooms
- 6 cups chopped kale
- 2 teaspoons Italian seasoning
- 10 eggs
- 2 cups milk
- 1 ½ cups shredded cheddar cheese divided

Instructions

1. Lightly oil a 9×13-inch baking dish and set bread cubes inside, set aside.

2. Add olive oil to a large sauté pan and set over medium heat. Add onion and ½ teaspoon salt and cook for 5 minutes. Add mushrooms and ½ teaspoon of pepper and cook for an additional 5 minutes. Add kale and Italian seasoning, and cook for 2 minutes, or until slightly wilted. Add vegetable mixture to the prepared pan with the bread and stir to gently distribute.

3. In a large bowl, whisk together eggs, milk, and remaining salt and pepper until well-blended. Add 1 cup cheddar cheese and stir to combine.

4. Pour the egg mixture over the bread and vegetables and sprinkle the remaining cheddar cheese, then cover tightly with foil. Let sit in the fridge overnight.

5. When ready to bake, preheat the oven to 350°F. Bake, tightly covered in foil, for 40 minutes. Uncover and bake for an additional 15 minutes, or until the center is puffy and the top is golden brown.

6. Let cool slightly before cutting into squares and serving.

2. Tortilla Wrap

Prep Time: 5 Minutes

Cook Time: 5 Minutes

Servings: 1

Ingredients

- 1 tablespoon butter plus more for greasing pan
- 2 eggs
- Dash sea salt
- 1 large burrito-sized tortilla
- ½ avocado mashed
- 2 tablespoons salsa
- 3 tablespoons shredded mozzarella cheese

Instructions

1. Place a burrito-sized tortilla on a flat service. Use scissors or a knife to make a cut from the bottom edge of the tortilla to the center.
2. Heat butter in nonstick skillet over medium-high heat. Whisk the eggs in small bowl, then carefully pour into the center of the pan. When the edges start

to set, start to gently fold the eggs until the eggs are cooked through, about 2-3 minutes.

3. With the tortilla slit made, imagine the tortilla made up of four quarters. Transfer the scrambled eggs to the bottom right quarter.

4. Add the mashed avocado to the second quarter, followed by the salsa in the third and the cheese in the fourth.

5. Starting with the bottom right quarter, fold the tortilla over the second quarter, then over the third quarter and finally, over the last quarter to form a triangle shape.

6. Transfer the tortilla to the same skillet or a grill pan with a little extra butter for greasing. Cook the tortilla on one side pressing down firmly with a flat spatula, until golden brown and crispy, about 2-3 minutes. Flip and cook on the other side for 2 more minutes until the cheese is melty and the edges are crisp.

7. Remove from heat and allow to rest for one minute before slicing in half.

3. Oatmeal Bars

Prep Time: 5 Minutes

Cook Time: 35 Minutes

Servings: 16

Ingredients

- 2 cups rolled oats
- ½ cup cane sugar
- 1 ½ teaspoons baking powder
- ½ teaspoon salt
- ½ teaspoon cinnamon
- 2 eggs
- ½ cup almond milk
- ¼ cup unsweetened applesauce
- 1 teaspoon vanilla extract
- ¼ cup walnuts finely chopped
- ¼ cup dried cranberries

Instructions

1. Preheat oven to 350°F. Line an 8-inch square pan with parchment paper hanging over the edge.

2. In a medium bowl, combine the dry ingredients including the rolled oats, sugar, baking powder, salt, and cinnamon together in a bowl.

3. In another large bowl, combine the wet ingredients including the eggs, milk, applesauce, and vanilla extract. Transfer the dry ingredients over the wet ingredients and set aside until flavors blend, about 20 minutes.

4. Fold in the walnuts and cranberries, and spread combined mixture into prepared square pan.

5. Bake in the preheated oven until edges are golden brown, about 30-35 minutes. Allow to cool on wire rack for 5 minutes before slicing. Cut into 16 bars.

4. Egg Cups

Prep Time: 5 Minutes

Cook Time: 15 Minutes

Servings: 3

Ingredients

- 6 large eggs
- Salt and pepper
- 1 cup baby spinach chopped
- ½ cup diced red peppers
- 2 tablespoons diced red onions
- ¼ cup shredded cheese

Instructions

1. Preheat the oven to 375°F. Coat a muffin tin with cooking spray or line six of the cups with paper liners.
2. Crack the eggs into a large bowl or measuring cup with spout, and use a whisk or hand blender to blend the eggs until smooth.
3. Add the spinach, peppers and onions into the greased muffin cup. Carefully pour the beaten eggs into each

of the six muffin cups until the liquid almost reaches the top. Season with salt and pepper. Sprinkle the cheese on top of each egg muffin

4. Bake for 15-18 minutes or until eggs are set.
5. Run a butter knife around the edges to help loosen them. Serve immediately.

5. Burritos

Prep Time: 15 Minutes

Cook Time: 12 Minutes

Servings: 4

Ingredients

- 1 tablespoon olive oil
- 1 red pepper seeded and diced
- ½ red onion diced
- Salt and pepper to taste
- 8 eggs
- ½ cup milk
- ½ cup prepared salsa
- Hot sauce to taste (optional)
- 1 ¼ cups shredded cheddar cheese divided
- 1 14.5 ounce can black beans drained and rinsed
- 4 large burrito size flour tortillas
- Nonstick spray as needed

1. In a large, nonstick skillet, heat olive oil over medium heat. Add red pepper and onion and season to taste with salt and pepper. Cook, stirring occasionally, for 5 minutes, or until the vegetables begin to soften.

2. Meanwhile, in a large bowl, combine eggs, milk, salsa, hot sauce (if using) and a pinch of salt and pepper. Whisk until smooth.

3. When the vegetables have softened, turn the heat to low and add egg mixture to the skillet. Cook, stirring constantly, until the eggs have cooked through, about 3 minutes.

4. Add 1 cup of cheddar cheese and the black beans and cook for 1 to 2 more minutes, or until cheese has melted. Remove egg mixture from heat and let cool slightly.

5. Once eggs have cooled, place a tortilla on a clean, dry surface. Add about 1 ½ cups of the egg mixture to the center of the tortilla. Starting at the bottom, fold the tortilla up and over the eggs, tucking the sides of the tortilla in as you roll. When there is one or two inches of tortilla remaining at the top, sprinkle about 1 tablespoon of the remaining grated cheese, then continue rolling so the seam with the cheese is on the

bottom of your surface. Repeat with remaining eggs and tortillas.

6. Spray a large nonstick skillet with cooking spray, then set over medium heat. Working with two burritos at a time, place them seam side down in the hot pan and cook for 1-2 minutes, or until the bottom is deeply golden brown. Remove from heat and repeat with remaining burritos.

7. If enjoying right away, cut in half and serve. If freezing for later use, let burritos cool completely, then wrap them tightly in foil and store in a large freezer-safe ziptop bag and place in the freezer for up to two months.

8. When ready to enjoy, you can reheat them two ways. To use the microwave, remove and discard foil and place on a microwave safe plate. Cover the burrito with a damp paper towel, then cook in the microwave for about 3 minutes. Cut in half to check if the burrito is heated through. If not, cover again with damp paper towel and heat for an additional 1-2 minutes. To reheat in an airfryer, remove and discard foil and place in an airfryer that has been preheated to 400°F. Cook for about 10-15 minutes, or until warm throughout. Note: After 10 minutes, cut the burrito in

half to check if it has been heated through. If not, cook until the inside is warm, about 5 more minutes.

6. Egg Wrap

Prep Time: 5 Minutes

Cook Time: 5 Minutes

Servings: 1

Ingredients

- 2 eggs
- 1 teaspoon water
- 1 teaspoon all-purpose flour
- Salt and pepper to taste
- 2 teaspoons olive oil

For the filling

- ½ avocado
- 1 teaspoon lemon juice
- ¼ teaspoon garlic powder
- 1 cup arugula
- 1 small tomato sliced
- 1 tablespoon feta cheese

Instructions

1. In a medium bowl, place the eggs, water, flour, salt and pepper; and whisk until well combined and the flour is completely dissolved.
2. Heat the olive oil in a nonstick frying pan over medium heat. Pour the egg mixture into the pan and spread it out evenly.
3. Cook for about 3 minutes until the egg mixture is completely set, breaking up any air bubbles that form. Gently slide a spatula under the edges of the egg mixture to flip. Slide the cooked egg wrap onto a plate to allow it to cool slightly.
4. To make the avocado spread, mash the avocado, garlic, lemon juice, salt and pepper in a small bowl.
5. Spread the mashed avocado over the entire egg wrap, top it with arugula, add sliced tomatoes and feta cheese. Roll it up tightly and then slice in half. Enjoy immediately!

7. Coffee Smoothie

Prep Time: 5 Minutes

Cook Time: 00 Minutes

Servings: 2

Ingredients

- 1 cup cold brewed coffee
- 1 ½ cup milk
- ¼ cup rolled oats
- 1 frozen banana
- 1 scoop vanilla protein
- 1 tablespoon cocoa powder
- ¼ teaspoon cinnamon

Instructions

1. Place all the ingredients in a high-speed blender, and blend for 60-120 seconds until you get a smooth and creamy texture.
2. Taste the smoothie, adding more milk if it is too thick or adding more sweetener if it's not sweet enough.

Pour into a cup or mason jar. Enjoy immediately, or store in the fridge for up to 24 hours.

8. Eggs & Sweet Potato Bowl

Prep Time: 5 Minutes

Cook Time: 25 Minutes

Servings: 1

Ingredients

- 1 large eggs
- 2 tablespoons olive oil divided
- 1 small sweet potato diced
- ½ teaspoon salt divided
- ½ teaspoon black pepper divided
- 1 garlic clove minced
- 3 cups kale leaves
- ⅛ teaspoon crushed red pepper
- ¼ ripe avocado sliced

Instructions

1. Place the egg in a small saucepan and submerge the egg with cool water. Bring the water to a boil uncovered. Turn off the heat, cover the pan and allow the egg to cook until soft boiled, 5 minutes. Transfer

the cooked egg to ice water to cool completely before peeling.

2. Meanwhile, heat 1 tablespoon olive oil in a large skillet over medium heat. Add the garlic and cook until fragrant, 1 minute. Add the kale and use tongs to toss with the olive oil and garlic. Season with ¼ teaspoon salt, ¼ teaspoon black pepper and crushed red pepper and cook until slightly wilted but still crisp, about 2 minutes. Transfer the kale to a bowl.

3. In the same skillet, add the remaining olive oil and the sweet potatoes and season with the remaining salt and pepper. Cook, stirring occasionally, until fork tender, about 15-20 minutes. Remove and add on top of the kale.

4. Cut the soft boiled egg in half and serve on top of the sweet potatoes and kale. Add the avocado and enjoy immediately.

9. English Muffin Pizza

Prep Time: 5 Minutes

Cook Time: 5 Minutes

Servings: 2

Ingredients

- 1 tablespoon butter
- 4 eggs
- ½ cup pizza sauce
- 2 whole-grain English muffins
- ½ cup shredded mozzarella cheese
- Sliced olives
- ¼ teaspoon oregano
- 1 tablespoon chopped basil
- Crushed red pepper optional

Instructions

1. Heat butter in nonstick skillet over medium-high heat until hot. Whisk the eggs in a small bowl, then carefully pour into the center of the pan. When the

edges start to set, start to gently fold the eggs until the eggs are cooked through, about 2-3 minutes.

2. Divide the eggs into 4 sides of whole grain English muffins. Layer pizza sauce on top, add shredded mozzarella and sliced olives and sprinkle with dried oregano.

3. Broil on high until the cheese melts, about 1-2 minutes. Top with fresh basil and crushed red pepper, and enjoy immediately.

10. Green Shakshuka

Prep Time: 10 Minutes

Cook Time: 20 Minutes

Servings: 3

Ingredients

- 2 tablespoons olive oil
- 1 cup onions sliced or diced
- 1 cup green bell peppers sliced or diced
- 2 garlic cloves minced
- 1/4 cup chopped cilantro plus more for garnish
- 1/2 teaspoon cumin
- 1 bunch kale destemmed, roughly chopped
- Salt and pepper
- 5 eggs
- 2 ounces feta cheese for serving
- Crusty bread for serving

Instructions

1. Preheat the oven to 375°F.

2. Heat olive oil in cast iron skillet over medium heat. Add the onions and peppers and cook for about 5 minutes until the onions become soft and translucent. Stir in garlic, cilantro and cumin, and cook for an additional 1-2 minutes until the garlic becomes fragrant.

3. Add the kale in batches, season with salt and pepper, and cook until they soften, but don't wilt, about 1-2 minutes. Turn off the heat. You can add ¼ cup water to soften the kale and create more of a sauce, but this is optional.

4. Using a wooden spoon or spatula, create 5 small nests between the vegetables. Gently crack the eggs into nests.

5. Transfer the skillet to the preheated oven and bake uncovered for 7-10 minutes, until the egg whites are set.

6. Remove the shakshuka from the oven and season with salt and pepper. Sprinkle feta cheese, garnish with cilantro, and serve with crusty bread, if desired.

LUNCH

11. Sweet Potato Hash with Eggs

Prep Time: 10 Minutes

Cook Time: 25 Minutes

Servings: 2

Ingredients

- 1 large sweet potato about ¾ pound, peeled and cut into ½-inch cubes
- 3 tablespoons avocado oil divided
- ½ teaspoon salt divided
- ½ teaspoon garlic powder
- ¼ teaspoon paprika
- ½ red onion diced
- 4 cups chopped kale tightly packed
- 4 eggs
- 2 tablespoons shredded parmesan cheese
- ¼ teaspoon crushed red pepper

1. Heat 2 tablespoons oil in a large skillet over medium heat. When the oil is almost smoking, add sweet potatoes, ¼ teaspoon salt, garlic powder and paprika. Toss sweet potatoes to evenly coat in the oil, then spread into a single layer and cook, undisturbed, until browned and crisp on the bottom. Flip potatoes and continue to cook until crispy all around, about 10-12 minutes in total. Remove to a small plate and set aside.

2. Add remaining 1 tablespoon oil and red onion to the pan. Cook until onion softens, 1-2 minutes, then add kale and remaining ¼ teaspoon salt. Cook until kale has wilted, about 2 minutes, then add sweet potatoes back in and toss to incorporate.

3. Make 4 evenly spaced wells in the hash and crack an egg into each. Cover the pan until egg whites are set and egg yolks are cooked to your desired doneness, 5-7 minutes . Top with parmesan cheese and red pepper flakes.

12. Avocado Toast with Egg

Prep Time: 3 Minutes

Cook Time: 7 Minutes

Servings: 1

Ingredients

- ¼ avocado seeded and peeled
- 1 slice whole grain bread or bread of choice
- Sea salt to taste
- Freshly cracked black pepper to taste
- Fried Eggs
- ½ tablespoon butter
- 1 large eggs
- Scrambled Eggs
- ½ tablespoon butter
- 2 eggs
- Boiled Eggs
- 2 eggs
- Poached Eggs
- 2 teaspoons white vinegar
- 1 large eggs

Instructions

1. Toast the bread in a toaster until golden and crispy, place the quarter avocado over the toast, slice it and mash it on top of the toast. Top with eggs of choice, and season with salt and pepper, to taste.
2. For fried eggs: Heat butter in nonstick skillet over medium-high heat until hot. Break the egg onto the skillet and immediately reduce the heat to low. Cook uncovered until whites are completely set and yolks are thickened to your liking, about 5-7 minutes.
3. For scrambled eggs: Heat butter in nonstick skillet over medium-high heat until hot. Whisk the eggs in small bowl, then carefully pour into the center of the pan. When the edges start to set, start to gently fold the eggs until the eggs are cooked through, about 2-3 minutes.
4. For boiled eggs: Place the eggs in a saucepan. Pour cool water over the eggs until fully submerged. Bring the water to a rolling boil, then reduce the heat to low and cook according to the desired doneness: 4 minutes for Soft boiled; 6 minutes for Medium boiled; 12 minutes for Hard boiled. Prepare a bowl of ice

water. Transfer the cooked eggs to the ice water to cool completely before peeling.

5. For poached eggs: Bring a large pot of water to a boil. Crack one egg into a small bowl. Stir vinegar into the water and create a vortex with the boiling water. Lower the heat so the water creates a rolling boil at the bottom of the pot. Then, carefully add the egg to the middle of the pot and cook for 3-4 minutes, according to desired doneness. Remove the egg with a slotted spoon.

13. Vegetable Frittata

Prep Time: 10 Minutes

Cook Time: 15 Minutes

Servings: 4

Ingredients

- 6 eggs
- ¼ cup whole milk yogurt
- 1 cup shredded mozzarella cheese divided
- ¼ cup red onions chopped
- 1 cup mushrooms chopped
- 8-10 stalks asparagus ends trimmed and chopped
- ¼ cup cilantro chopped
- ½ cup cherry tomatoes sliced

Instructions

1. Preheat the oven to 425° degrees.
2. Whisk together the egg, yogurt, half the shredded mozzarella cheese and salt & pepper; set mixture aside.

3. Heat olive oil in an oven safe pan or cast iron pan. Add onions, mushrooms and asparagus and cook for 3-5 minutes until the vegetables soften.

4. Pour the egg mixture on top of the cooked vegetables. Place sliced cherry tomatoes on top and add the remaining cheese.

5. Bake uncovered in the preheated oven until the center is set, and not jiggly, about 10-15 minutes

14. Quinoa Avocado Salad

Prep Time: 15 Minutes

Cook Time: 20 Minutes

Servings: 6

Ingredients

- 1 cup uncooked quinoa
- 1 cup grape tomatoes halved
- 1 large cucumber diced
- ¼ cup red onion finely chopped
- 2 large ripe avocados chopped
- ¼ cup chopped cilantro

Dressing

- 1/4 cup olive oil
- 1 tablespoon red wine vinegar
- 1 tablespoon lime juice
- 1 teaspoon Dijon mustard
- 1 garlic clove minced
- ½ teaspoon salt

Instructions

1. Place the quinoa in a medium sauce pan over medium heat. Toast without oil or salt for 5-7 minutes until the seeds start to pop and become aromatic. Add 2 cups of water to the quinoa and bring to a boil, then turn down the heat to low. Cover and simmer the quinoa for 15 minutes. Remove from the heat and keep covered for an additional 10 minutes. Fluff with a fork and season with salt.

2. To make the dressing, whisk together the olive oil, red wine vinegar, lime juice, Dijon mustard, garlic and salt.

3. When the quinoa is cool, place it in a bowl and add all the ingredients for the salad on top. Pour the dressing on top and stir gently to combine. Serve at room temperature or chilled.

15. Roasted Vegetable Grilled Cheese Sandwich

Prep Time: 5 Minutes

Cook Time: 20 Minutes

Servings: 2

Ingredients

- 1 zucchini sliced
- 1 yellow squash sliced
- 1 eggplant sliced
- 1 red pepper sliced
- ¼ cup red onions sliced
- Olive oil spray
- ½ teaspoon dill
- Salt and pepper to taste
- 2 tablespoons butter
- 4 slices thick bread
- 4 ounces Dill Havarti cheese divided
- 4 ounces Gouda cheese divided

Instructions

1. Preheat oven to 400°F. Toss the vegetables with olive oil spray and dill and season with salt and pepper. Spread out on a baking sheet and roast for 10 minutes, until vegetables are slightly tender.

2. Brush the melted butter on one side of the bread slices.

3. In a large cast iron skillet or electric griddle over medium low heat, place one slice of bread on the skillet, buttered side down. Add half the Dill Havarti cheese on top of the bread, then layer with half the roasted vegetables, followed by half the Gouda cheese. Top with a bread slice, buttered side up.

4. Cook grilled cheese sandwich until golden brown and cheese is melted, about 4-6 minutes on each side. Repeat for the second sandwich.

16. Avocado Egg Salad

Prep Time: 10 Minutes

Cook Time: 10 Minutes

Servings: 4

Ingredients

- 4 eggs
- 2 tablespoons Greek yogurt
- 1 tablespoon lemon juice
- 1 teaspoon Dijon mustard
- Salt and pepper to taste
- 1 avocado pitted and peeled
- 1 teaspoon chives
- Sliced bread for sandwich
- Lettuce for sandwich

Instructions

1. Place cold eggs into boiling hot water. Boil on medium for 12 minutes. Use a slotted spoon to remove the eggs from the boiling water. Place in an ice bath, then remove, peel and chop the eggs roughly

2. To make the dressing, combine the Greek yogurt, lemon juice and Dijon mustard. Season with salt and pepper and whisk to combine.

3. Add the avocado on top of the dressing and toss to combine. Then mash with a fork until it's creamy. Add the hard-boiled eggs and combine once more.

4. Serve in a sandwich with bread of choice and lettuce, if desired.

17. Mediterranean White Bean Soup

Prep Time: 10 Minutes

Cook Time: 25 Minutes

Servings: 6

Ingredients

- 1 tablespoon olive oil
- 1 large onion chopped
- 2 garlic cloves minced
- 2-3 large carrots chopped
- 2-3 celery stalks chopped
- 6 cups vegetable broth
- 1 teaspoon dried thyme
- ½ teaspoon oregano
- 1 teaspoon salt
- ½ teaspoon black pepper
- 3 15-ounces canned white beans drained and rinsed
- 2 cups baby spinach
- Fresh parsley finely chopped, for serving
- Grated parmesan cheese for serving

Instructions

1. In a large pot or saucepan, heat olive over medium high heat. Add onions and cook until onions are translucent, about 3-5 minutes. Add the garlic, carrots, celery, thyme, oregano, salt and pepper, and cook for an additional 2-3 minutes.
2. Add vegetable broth and beans, bring to a boil, reduce heat and simmer for 15 minutes to combine all of the flavors together.
3. Stir in the spinach and continue to simmer until the spinach wilts, about 2 minutes
4. Remove from heat, sprinkle fresh parsley and grated parmesan cheese, if desired, and serve immediately.

18. Roasted Vegetable Grilled Cheese Sandwich

Prep Time: 5 Minutes

Cook Time: 20 Minutes

Servings: 2

Ingredients

- 1 zucchini sliced
- 1 yellow squash sliced
- 1 eggplant sliced
- 1 red pepper sliced
- ¼ cup red onions sliced
- Olive oil spray
- ½ teaspoon dill
- Salt and pepper to taste
- 2 tablespoons butter
- 4 slices thick bread
- 4 ounces Dill Havarti cheese divided
- 4 ounces Gouda cheese divided

Instructions

1. Preheat oven to 400°F. Toss the vegetables with olive oil spray and dill and season with salt and pepper. Spread out on a baking sheet and roast for 10 minutes, until vegetables are slightly tender.

2. Brush the melted butter on one side of the bread slices.

3. In a large cast iron skillet or electric griddle over medium low heat, place one slice of bread on the skillet, buttered side down. Add half the Dill Havarti cheese on top of the bread, then layer with half the roasted vegetables, followed by half the Gouda cheese. Top with a bread slice, buttered side up.

4. Cook grilled cheese sandwich until golden brown and cheese is melted, about 4-6 minutes on each side. Repeat for the second sandwich.

19. Turkey Panini

Prep Time: 2 Minutes

Cook Time: 2 Minutes

Servings: 1

Ingredients

- 3 ounces sourdough bread 2 slices sliced about ½ inch thick
- 1 tablespoon mayonnaise
- 3 ounces turkey breast
- 2 tablespoons cranberry sauce
- 1 slice provolone cheese
- 1 tablespoon fresh thyme

Instructions

1. Heat a panini press or skillet to medium high heat.
2. Spread the mayonnaise on both sides of the bread. Lay the slices down on a clean work surface. Place the sliced turkey breast on top of one slice of bread. Add the fresh thyme leaves, then the cranberry sauce and finally the provolone cheese.

3. Cover the sandwich with the other slice of bread.

4. Transfer the sandwich to a panini press or hot skillet.
    Press together gently to help the whole sandwich stick
    together. Cook it until the bread is crisp and golden
    and the cheese is melted, about 3-4 minutes.

5. Slice the sandwich in half and serve immediately.

20. Mediterranean White Bean Soup

Prep Time: 10 Minutes

Cook Time: 25 Minutes

Servings: 6

Ingredients

- 1 tablespoon olive oil
- 1 large onion chopped
- 2 garlic cloves minced
- 2-3 large carrots chopped
- 2-3 celery stalks chopped
- 6 cups vegetable broth
- 1 teaspoon dried thyme
- ½ teaspoon oregano
- 1 teaspoon salt
- ½ teaspoon black pepper
- 3 15-ounces canned white beans drained and rinsed
- 2 cups baby spinach
- Fresh parsley finely chopped, for serving
- Grated parmesan cheese for serving

Instructions

1. In a large pot or saucepan, heat olive over medium high heat. Add onions and cook until onions are translucent, about 3-5 minutes. Add the garlic, carrots, celery, thyme, oregano, salt and pepper, and cook for an additional 2-3 minutes.
2. Add vegetable broth and beans, bring to a boil, reduce heat and simmer for 15 minutes to combine all of the flavors together.
3. Stir in the spinach and continue to simmer until the spinach wilts, about 2 minutes
4. Remove from heat, sprinkle fresh parsley and grated parmesan cheese, if desired, and serve immediately.

DINNER

21. Pinwheel Sandwiches – 4 ways

Prep Time: 10 Minutes

Cook Time: 00 Minutes

Servings: 4

Ingredients

Hummus & Veggies

- 2 large burrito-size tortillas
- ¼ cup prepared hummus
- 1 carrot peeled into ribbons
- 1 small zucchini peeled into ribbons
- 1 small red pepper cut into matchsticks
- Everything Bagel Cucumber & Tomato
- 2 large burrito-size tortillas
- 2 tablespoons cream cheese at room temperature
- 2 teaspoons everything bagel seasoning
- 2 small Persian cucumbers shaved into ribbons
- 1 small tomato thinly sliced (you'll want about 6 slices)
- Pesto Turkey

- 2 large burrito-size tortillas
- 2 tablespoons prepared pesto
- 6 thin slices of deli style turkey breast
- 6 thin slices cheddar cheese
- 1 cup loosely packed baby spinach
- Chicken Salad
- 2 large burrito-size tortillas
- 8 butter lettuce leaves
- 1 cup shredded cooked chicken
- ¼ cup Greek yogurt
- ½ lemon juiced
- 1 tablespoon chopped dill
- 2 teaspoons Dijon mustard
- 1 celery stalk diced
- Salt and pepper to taste

Instructions

1. For the first three pinwheels: Place the tortillas on a large cutting board. Add the spreadable ingredient (hummus, cream cheese or pesto to each tortilla, spreading into an even layer all over the surface of the tortilla.

2. Divide any of the remaining ingredients evenly between each tortilla, layering them in the center of the tortilla.

3. For the chicken salad pinwheel: Place the tortillas on a large cutting board. Add four leaves of butter lettuce to each tortilla. In a medium bowl, combine chicken, Greek yogurt, lemon juice, dill, Dijon, celery, salt and pepper. Stir until all of the chicken is evenly coated with the yogurt mixture. Add half of the prepared chicken salad on top of each, spreading it into an even layer.

4. To roll the pinwheels: Take the bottom portion of the tortilla, and fold it about ⅔ of the way up and over the vegetables. Using your fingers, pull back on the folded over portion of the tortilla to create the start of a tight spiral.

22. Roasted Vegetable Grilled Cheese Sandwich

Prep Time: 5 Minutes

Cook Time: 20 Minutes

Servings: 2

Ingredients

- 1 zucchini sliced
- 1 yellow squash sliced
- 1 eggplant sliced
- 1 red pepper sliced
- ¼ cup red onions sliced
- Olive oil spray
- ½ teaspoon dill
- Salt and pepper to taste
- 2 tablespoons butter
- 4 slices thick bread
- 4 ounces Dill Havarti cheese divided
- 4 ounces Gouda cheese divided

Instructions

1. Preheat oven to 400°F. Toss the vegetables with olive oil spray and dill and season with salt and pepper. Spread out on a baking sheet and roast for 10 minutes, until vegetables are slightly tender.

2. Brush the melted butter on one side of the bread slices.

3. In a large cast iron skillet or electric griddle over medium low heat, place one slice of bread on the skillet, buttered side down. Add half the Dill Havarti cheese on top of the bread, then layer with half the roasted vegetables, followed by half the Gouda cheese. Top with a bread slice, buttered side up.

4. Cook grilled cheese sandwich until golden brown and cheese is melted, about 4-6 minutes on each side. Repeat for the second sandwich.

23. Butternut squash soup

Prep Time: 15 Minutes

Cook Time: 55 Minutes

Servings: 6

Ingredients

Soup

- 2 medium butternut squash (approx. 6 cups) peeled, seeds removed and chopped into equal sized chunks
- 4-5 garlic cloves peeled and chopped
- olive oil extra virgin
- salt & fresh ground pepper
- 1 large white or yellow onion
- 1/4 tsp red pepper flakes
- 1/2 tsp salt
- 1 1/2 tsp ginger freshly grated or paste
- 1/2 tsp fresh thyme chopped
- 3 cups water or vegetable broth
- 1 cup almond milk unsweetened
- juice of two limes

Shiitake Bacon

- 1 pound shiitake mushrooms trimmed and thinly sliced
- 1/4 cup olive oil extra virgin
- 1 1/4 tsp salt
- 1/2 tsp fresh ground pepper

Macadamia Nut Sour Cream

- 1 cup macadamia nuts soaked in warm water for 1 hour
- 1 tbsp lemon juice fresh squeezed
- 1/2 tsp salt or to taste

Instructions

Soup Instructions:

1. Preheat. oven to 400°.
2. Prepare. To prepare the squash for roasting, trim off both ends of each butternut squash, then cut through where the neck meets the bulb. (This makes it easier to peel.) Peel both pieces of squash with a vegetable peeler. Cut squash neck and bulb in half lengthwise. Using a spoon, scoop out seeds from each half of the bulb; discard seeds. Place squash pieces cut side down on board and cut each piece in half lengthwise. Cut

squash crosswise into 1"-thick slices. You don't need to worry about beautiful knife work here, but it's good for the pieces to be similarly sized so they cook at the same rate.

3. Roast. On two sheet pans lined with parchment paper, add your butternut squash pieces and garlic cloves (skins removed). Drizzle olive oil over squash, add salt & fresh ground pepper and give them a good mix to make sure the oil is distributed evenly. Place both pans in the oven and Roast for 30-35 minutes, stirring once or twice, cooking until squash is fork tender. Remove any garlic that seem to be over roasting and set aside. Once done, remove and let cool for 10 to 15 min.

4. Saute. In the meantime while squash and garlic is roasting. Heat 2 Tbsp. oil in a large Dutch oven or saucepan over medium heat. Add onions, ¼ tsp. red pepper flakes, and 1 tsp salt, sauté until onion is translucent and soft, 4–5 minutes. Add ginger, 1/2 teaspoon fresh thyme and sauté another 1-2 minutes. turn off heat and set aside.

5. Combine. Time to combine your squash and garlic to the onion mixture, add 3 cups water, or enough to just submerge the squash, and 1 cup of almond milk, add

some salt, then stir to combine. Raise heat to high and bring soup to a boil. Once soup is boiling, reduce heat to medium-low and simmer, stirring occasionally, 10-15 minutes.

6. Blend. Set up your workstation. You'll need your pot of soup, blender, a large bowl, a ladle, and a clean kitchen towel all within arm's reach. Using ladle, fill blender pitcher no more than halfway with equal parts broth and vegetables (don't fill it up, it will overflow as it blends!). Secure the blender lid, cover with a folded kitchen towel and hold down, start out blending on a low setting and then increase until soup becomes smooth. Slowly remove lid away from you to let steam escape (many blender lids come with removable vents). Transfer to a large bowl. Repeat, working in batches, until all soup is blended.

7. Transfer. Transfer soup back to your dutch oven on the stove top and cook over medium heat Stir in lime juice. Taste and add more salt & fresh ground pepper if needed.

8. Serve. Ladle soup into bowls. Top with Make Ahead garnishes (see below) serve and enjoy. Pictured. I garnished with macadamia nut cream, shiitake bacon,

toasted pumpkin seeds and extra fresh thyme, red pepper, black pepper and a lime wedge.

9. Make-Ahead. Shiitake Bacon Directions:

10. Preheat. Preheat the oven to 375°F.

11. Cook. On a large rimmed baking sheet, toss mushrooms with oil, salt, and pepper. Bake for about 30 minutes, turning frequently with a spatula, until lightly browned and crisp.

12. Cool. Shiitake bacon will crisp more when cooled.

Make-Ahead. Macadamia Nut Sour Cream:

1. Soak. Soak nuts in warm water for 1 hour. Drain and rinse.Combine. Combine macadamia nuts, lemon juice, salt and water if needed in a high speed blender until smooth.

24. Lentil Loaf

Prep Time: 30 Minutes

Cook Time: 1hr 30 Minutes

Servings: 6

Ingredients

Lentils

- 1 cup French lentils soaked overnight
- 1/2 cup red lentils soaked overnight
- 1 bay leaf
- 3-4 cups water

Dry Ingredients

- 1 1/2 cup quick oats processed
- 1 tbsp Italian seasoning
- 1 tbsp cumin
- 1/2 tbsp thyme
- 1/2 tbsp onion powder
- salt & pepper to taste

Vegetable Mixture

- 1 tbsp neutral oil

- 1 lg white onion finely minced
- 1 tsp salt
- 2 cloves garlic finely minced
- 1 lg carrot peeled, finely chopped
- 2 celery stocks finely chopped
- 1 red pepper seeds removed, finely chopped
- 1/2 cup shiitake mushrooms finely chopped
- 2 tbsp tomato paste double concentrate
- 1 cup vegetable stock

Flax Egg

- 3 tbsp flax ground
- 6 tbsp water

Glaze

- 5 tbsp ketchup
- 1 1/2 tbsp nutritional yeast
- 1 tbsp maple syrup
- 1/2 tbsp balsamic vinegar

Garnish (Optional)

- fresh Italian parsley finely chopped

Instructions

Lentils

2. Night Before. Soak. In a medium-size bowl, cover lentils in at least 3 inches of water and soak overnight.

3. Rinse. Rinse and drain.

4. Cook. In a medium saucepan, combine lentils, bay leaf and 3-4 cups of water and bring to a boil. Once boiling turn heat down to simmer and let cook until lentils become soft about 25-30 minutes.

5. Drain. Drain set aside to cool.

Dry Ingredients

1. Process. In a highspeed blender or food processor, process oats until fine.

2. Combine. In a large bowl, combine processed oats, Italian seasoning, cumin, thyme, onion powder, salt & pepper and mix well. Set aside.

Vegetable Mixture

1. Saute. Heat a large skillet with 1 tablespoon neutral oil on medium-high heat. Add onions and a generous pinch of salt and saute until translucent about 1-2 minutes, add garlic and saute until garlic becomes fragrant. Add. Shiitake mushrooms, carrot, celery, red pepper, tomato paste and stir to combine. Add. Vegetable stock and turn heat to medium-low and

cover. Let cook stirring occasionally until mushrooms have released their liquid, vegetables have softened and most of the cooking liquid has absorbed, about 20 minutes. Remove lid and cook a few more minutes until all liquid is absorbed. Turn off heat set aside and let cool.

Flax Egg And Glaze

2. Meanwhile, while the vegetables are cooking. Preheat. The oven to 375 degrees Fahrenheit.

Prepare. Flax egg and glaze.

3. Flax Egg. In a small bowl, combine ground flax and water and stir well to incorporate and let it soak for up to 15 minutes. The flax will expand and congeal. This will be our binding agent that keeps the lentil loaf intact.

4. Glaze. In a small bowl, combine ketchup, nutritional yeast, balsamic vinegar, and maple syrup. Stir well to combine.

Bring It All Together

1. Combine. In the large bowl, containing the dry ingredients add cooled lentils, vegetable mixture, and flax egg. Using your hands blend all ingredients

together until well combined and dough like. This is a good time to taste and adjust seasonings.

2. Cook. Transfer dough to a lightly oiled or (if removing meatloaf to put on serving dish) parchment lined meatloaf pan.

3. Glaze. Brush glaze mixture on top of the lentil loaf covering all edges of the loaf.

4. Cover & Bake. Cover with tin foil and bake for 45 minutes. Remove tin foil and bake another 5-10 minutes uncovered.

5. Remove. Remove from oven and let cool and rest for 15 minutes. The meatloaf will cut better.

Garnish

1. Garnish is optional. I like to add fresh Italian (flat-leaf) parsley down the middle for a burst of color and some added flavor.

25. Martha's guacamole

Prep Time: 15 Minutes

Cook Time: 00 Minutes

Servings: 6

Ingredients

- 3 lg avocados peeled, and pit removed
- 1/4 onion minced
- 1 jalapeño seeds removed, minced
- 1 1/2 bunch cilantro finely chopped
- 1 lime juiced
- salt to taste

Instructions

1. Place the onion and jalapeno in the mortar (bowl) and use the pestle to crush them as best you can.
2. Add in the avocados and mash until you get a consistency you like.
3. Stir in the cilantro, lime juice, and salt.
4. Serve.

26. Papaspicosas (Spicy Potato Tacos)

Prep Time: 20 Minutes

Cook Time: 35 Minutes

Servings: 8

Ingredients

Potato Filling

- 1/4 cup grape-seed oil
- 6 large yellow potatoes peeled and cut into 1-inch pieces
- 1 yellow onion diced
- 3 cloves garlic thinly sliced
- 2 cups vegetable broth
- 4 fresh jalapeños halved and seeded
- 1 teaspoon oregano preferably Mexican
- 1 teaspoon cumin
- 1/3 cup fresh cilantro
- 1/4 teaspoon salt or to taste

Tacos

- 8-10 corn tortillas warmed
- sliced green onions

- cilantro
- cabbage or lettuce thinly sliced
- toasted pepitas
- cashew sour cream or store bought

Instructions

 Taco Filling

Cook. In an extra large skillet, heat oil over medium-high heat. Add potatoes. Cook 10 minutes, turning occasionally and adding chopped onion and garlic the last 5 minutes.

Blend. While the potatoes are cooking, warm vegetable broth and transfer to a blender. Add chili peppers, oregano, cumin, cilantro and salt. Blend until smooth.

Combine. Add broth mixture to potatoes in the extra large skillet. Simmer uncovered for 15 minutes or until potatoes are tender and liquid reaches a thick sauce like consistency. Lower heat and cover the pan for another 10 minutes, stirring occasionally.

27. Asparagus Soup

Prep Time: 20 Minutes

Cook Time: 30 Minutes

Servings: 4

Ingredients

- 1-2 tablespoon vegetable broth or water
- 4 cups asparagus ends trimmed and chopped (approx 1 bunch)
- 1 yellow onion thinly sliced
- 3 garlic cloves minced
- 2 yukon gold potatoes peeled and chopped
- 4 cups vegetable broth
- 1 bay leaf
- juice of 1 lemon
- salt & pepper to taste
- Optional toppings
- toasted black sesame seeds
- red pepper flakes
- lightly steamed asparagus tips
- fresh ground pepper
- extra lemon juice

Instructions

1. Prep. Clean, peel, and chop onion, garlic, potatoes, and asparagus.

2. Saute. Set instant pot on sauté mode and add 1-2 tablespoons vegetable broth or water and heat on medium heat. Once warm, add chopped onions and a pinch of salt and sauté until onions become translucent, about 2 min. Then add garlic and sauté until it becomes fragrant.

3. Add. Add the vegetable broth, bay leaf, asparagus, potatoes, salt & pepper. Give it a good stir.

4. Pressure. Attach pressure cooker's lid and change settings to high pressure for 17 minutes. The pressure cooker will have to take a few minutes to build up pressure before the timer starts.

5. Natural Release. After 17 minutes and the timer goes off, allow the pressure cooker to naturally release its pressure by simply doing nothing to it for 8-10 minutes. After 8-10 minutes, turn the steam release knob on top of the lid to expel any remaining pressure.

6. Add. Squeeze in juice of 1 lemon.

7. Blend. Transfer soup to a high-speed blender. You may have to do it in batches. Make sure your blender lid is on tight. I place a dish towel on top of the lid, before blending to ensure I don't burn myself, if by chance the lid is loose.

8. Adjust. Taste and adjust seasonings to your liking.

9. Garnish & Serve.

28. 7 layer Mexican salad

Prep Time: 40 Minutes

Cook Time: 00 Minutes

Servings: 12

Ingredients

- 4 organic corn tortillas cut into strips
- 2 cups organic corn frozen or canned
- 6 cups romaine lettuce chopped
- 4 roma tomatoes chopped
- 1 15-oz can black beans rinsed and drained
- 1 15-oz can pinto. beans rinsed and drained
- 2 avocados halved, seeded, peeled and chopped
- 1 bunch fresh cilantro finely chopped

Lime Sour Cream

- 1 block silken tofu drained
- 1/4 cup olive oil extra virgin
- 1 lg lime juiced
- 1/2 tsp sea salt

Dressing

- 1 jar salsa

Instructions

Crunchy Corn Strips

1. Preheat oven to 400 degrees. Place tortilla strips in a shallow baking pan. Bake 8-10 minutes stirring occasionally, until strips are lightly browned and crisped. Remove from oven and let cool. They will crisp more upon cooling.

Lime Sour Cream

2. Blend. In a high-speed, blender add silken tofu, olive oil, lime juice, and salt and blend until smooth. Add a small amount of water if needed to acquire desired consistency. Set aside.

Layered Salad

3. Layer. In a 4-qt. Glass bowl layer ingredients starting with chopped romaine then tomatoes, black beans, corn, pinto beans, cilantro, and avocado.
4. Top. Spread lime sour cream evenly across the top of the layered salad, add crunchy corn strips and serve with salsa to dress.

29. Vegan mac n cheese with shiitake bacon

Prep Time: 15 Minutes

Cook Time: 30 Minutes

Servings: 4

Ingredients

- 1 tablespoon vegan butter I use miyokos
- 2 cups unsweetened almond milk
- 1 cup nutritional yeast
- 2 cups raw cashews soaked overnight
- juice of one small lemon
- 1 tablespoon garlic powder
- 1 tablespoon onion powder
- 1 teaspoon salt or to taste
- 1/2 turmeric powder
- smoked paprika for garnish (optional
- chives finely minced for garnish (optional)
- Shiitake bacon for garnish optional
- Shiitake bacon
- 1 pound shiitake mushrooms stemmed and sliced ¼ in thick

- ¼ cup grapeseed oil or other cold pressed vegetable oil
- 1¼ tsp fine sea salt
- freshly ground black pepper

Instructions

1. Soak. Soak raw cashews covered in water overnight on countertop covered with a. dish towel.
2. Blend. Add cashews, almond milk, lemon juice and seasonings to a blender and blend until smooth.
3. Adjust. Taste and adjust seasonings if desired.
4. Heat. Transfer Cheese sauce to a medium saucepan and heat on medium low heat. Until warmed.
5. Pour. The cheese sauce over your choice of pasta and stir to incorporate.
6. Garnish. Garnish with smoked paprika, shiitake bacon, chives and serve immediately.
7. Enjoy!
8. Shiitake mushrooms
9. Preheat. Preheat oven to 375 degrees.
10. Meanwhile. In a large bowl, toss sliced mushrooms with sunflower oil, sea salt, and freshly ground pepper. Allow to marinate 30 minutes before cooking.

11. Line. Line a baking sheet with parchment paper. Layout shiitake mushrooms in a single layer on baking sheet and bake for about 30 minutes, until steam disappears and the shiitakes are evenly browned.They will shrink considerably.

12. Cool. Remove the mushrooms and allow to cool, mushrooms will crisp as they cool.

30. Lemony Pea Spread with Pita Chips

Prep Time: 20 Minutes

Cook Time: 15 Minutes

Servings: 25

Ingredients

Pea Mash

- 2 garlic cloves quartered
- 1/2 cup fresh flat leaf parsley leaves
- 2 tablespoons extra virgin olive oil divided
- 1/2 cup water
- salt to taste
- 2 15- oz cans organic peas
- 4 tablespoons fresh chives chopped
- 2 tablespoons finely chopped preserved lemon peel divided Preserved lemons
- 2 tablespoons fresh lemon juice
- 1/2 teaspoon Aleppo pepper or crushed red pepper flakes plus more for serving
- freshly ground pepper

Pita Chips

- 4 pita bread rounds

- 1/2 cup vegan butter melted

- garlic powder

- salt to taste

Instructions

Pea Mash

1. Combine. In a saucepan, combine garlic, parsley, 1
   tablespoon oil, a pinch of salt and 1/2 cup water.
2. Cook. Add peas and cook over medium heat, stirring
   to combine the flavors for about 3-4 minutes.
3. Drain. Drain extra cooking fluid into a small bowl to
   use later in the recipe.
4. Tranfer. Transfer pea mixture to high speed blender
   or food processor and pulse until a coarse paste
   forms.Transfer to medium bowl, then mix in chives, 1
   tablespoon preserved lemon peel, 1 tablespoon lemon
   juice, 1/4 teaspoon Aleppo pepper, and 1 tablespoon
   oil.
5. Stir. Stir in saved cooking liquid, one tablespoon at a
   time, until mixture is still a thick consistency, but
   spreadable.
6. Season. Season pea spread with additional salt, black
   pepper, and more lemon juice, if desired.
7. Spread. Spread the pea mixture on each pita chip,
   sprinkle with remaining lemon peel, additional
   Aleppo pepper and drizzle with remaining oil, if
   desired.

8. Garnish. Garnish with fresh chopped herbs or edible flowers.

9. Enjoy!

Pita Chips

1. Preheat. Preheat oven to 400 degrees.

2. Prep. Cut around the edges of the pita rounds with a kitchen knife or scissors and separate. With a pizza cutter or scissors to desired shape and size.

3. Spread. Place the pita chips on a baking pan and spread the melted vegan butter on the rough side of each pita chip.

4. Sprinkle. Sprinkle garlic powder and salt over each piece. I also like to add more Aleppo pepper.

5. Cook. Cook the pita chips until lightly browned, for approximately 15 minutes. They should be just slightly crispy when you take them, as they crisp more when out of the oven.